LIVING A HEALTHY LIFE STYLE

VICTOR ONUZURU

DEDICATION

DEDICATED TO YOU

Contents

ACKNOWLEDGMENTS

I would like to express my deepest gratitude to all those who have contributed to the creation of this book. First and foremost, I would like to thank my family and friends for their unwavering support and encouragement throughout this journey.

I would also like to thank the team at the publisher for their guidance and expertise in bringing this book to fruition. Additionally, I would like to extend my appreciation to the researchers and experts whose work has informed the content of this book.

Finally, I am grateful to the readers who have chosen to invest their time and energy into reading this book. It is my hope that the information and insights presented here will be of value to you in your pursuit of a healthier lifestyle.

CHAPTER 1

The Importance of Living a Healthy Lifestyle

Living a healthy lifestyle is critical for preventing chronic diseases such as diabetes, heart disease, and cancer. It can also improve mental health, boost energy levels, and enhance overall quality of life. By adopting healthy habits, you can reduce the risk of developing these diseases and live a longer, happier life.

CHAPTER 2

A healthy diet is one of the most critical components of a healthy lifestyle. It should be rich in whole foods such as fruits, vegetables, whole grains, and lean protein sources. Limiting processed foods, added sugars, and unhealthy fats is also important for maintaining a healthy weight and reducing the risk of chronic diseases.

CHAPTER 3

Physical activity is essential for maintaining a healthy weight, reducing the risk of chronic diseases, and improving overall physical health. It is recommended that adults engage in at least 150 minutes of moderate-intensity aerobic exercise or 75 minutes of vigorous-intensity aerobic exercise each week. Strength training is also beneficial for building muscle and maintaining bone density.

Getting enough sleep is crucial for overall health and well-being. Sleep deprivation can lead to a range of health problems, including obesity, diabetes, and heart disease. Adults should aim for 7-8 hours of sleep each night, and establish a regular sleep schedule to promote healthy sleep habits.

Stress can have a significant impact on both physical and mental health. Chronic stress can lead to a range of health problems, including anxiety, depression, and heart disease. Finding healthy ways to manage stress, such as exercise, meditation, or deep breathing, is essential for maintaining overall health and well-being.

CHAPTER 6

Maintaining healthy relationships and social connections is crucial for overall well-being. Studies have shown that social isolation can increase the risk of chronic diseases and mental health problems. Making time for friends and family and engaging in social activities can help promote a sense of belonging and enhance overall quality of life.

CHAPTER 7

Alcohol and tobacco use can have a significant impact on overall health and well-being. Excessive alcohol consumption can lead to liver disease, cancer, and other health problems. Smoking is a leading cause of lung cancer and can increase the risk of heart disease and stroke. Limiting alcohol and tobacco use or quitting altogether is essential for maintaining a healthy lifestyle.

Regular medical care is essential for maintaining overall health and well-being. It allows for early detection and treatment of chronic diseases and other health problems. It is recommended that adults receive regular check-ups and screenings for various health conditions.

Incorporating healthy habits into daily life can be challenging, but it is essential for maintaining a healthy lifestyle. Small changes such as taking the stairs instead of the elevator, packing a healthy lunch, or going for a walk during lunch break can make a significant difference in overall health and well-being.

CHAPTER 10

Many barriers can prevent individuals from living a healthy lifestyle. These barriers include lack of time, motivation, or knowledge about healthy habits. Finding practical ways to overcome these barriers, such as setting realistic goals and seeking support from friends and family, can help individuals adopt healthy habits and live a healthier life.here.

In conclusion, living a healthy lifestyle is essential for achieving optimal health and well-being. It involves making conscious choices about diet, physical activity, sleep, stress management, social connections, alcohol and tobacco use, and regular medical care. By incorporating healthy habits into daily life, individuals can reduce the risk of chronic diseases and improve their quality of life.

Living a healthy lifestyle may seem challenging at first, but it is achievable with small changes and consistency over time. It is essential to set realistic goals and find ways to overcome any barriers that may prevent individuals from adopting healthy habits. Seeking support from friends, family, or a healthcare professional can also help individuals stay on track and achieve their health goals.

It is never too late to start living a healthy lifestyle. Even small changes, such as choosing whole foods over processed foods, taking a daily walk, or practicing stress management techniques, can make a significant difference in overall health and well-being. By prioritizing health and making conscious choices, individuals can live a healthier, happier life.

Here are some additional tips to help individuals live a healthy lifestyle:

Stay hydrated: Drinking plenty of water throughout the day is essential for maintaining good health. Water helps to regulate body temperature, transport nutrients and oxygen to cells, and remove waste products from the body.

Practice mindful eating: Mindful eating involves paying attention to the food you are eating, savoring each bite, and tuning into your body's hunger and fullness signals. This can help individuals make healthier food choices and avoid overeating.

Reduce screen time: Spending too much time in front of screens, whether it's a computer, TV, or phone, can lead to eye strain, headaches, and disrupted sleep patterns. Limiting screen time and taking regular breaks can help individuals reduce these negative effects.

Practice self-care: Taking time for self-care activities, such as reading, taking a bath, or practicing meditation, can help individuals reduce stress and improve mental health.

Connect with nature: Spending time in nature, whether it's a walk in the park or a hike in the woods, can help individuals reduce stress, improve mood, and promote physical activity.

Living a healthy lifestyle is a journey, not a destination. It involves making a commitment to prioritize health and well-being, and taking small steps every day to achieve these goals. With time, patience, and consistency, individuals can live a healthier, happier life and reduce the risk of chronic diseases.

Get enough sleep: Sleep plays a critical role in overall health and well-being. Getting enough sleep is essential for maintaining healthy brain function, regulating mood, and reducing the risk of chronic diseases such as heart disease and diabetes. Most adults need between 7-9 hours of sleep per night, but this can vary depending on individual needs.

Practice stress management: Chronic stress can have negative effects on both physical and mental health. Practicing stress management techniques such as meditation, deep breathing, or yoga can help individuals reduce stress and improve overall well-being.

Make time for physical activity: Regular physical activity is essential for maintaining good health. It can help individuals maintain a healthy weight, reduce the risk of chronic diseases, and improve mood and energy levels. Aim for at least 30 minutes of moderate-intensity physical activity, such as brisk walking or cycling, most days of the week.

Limit alcohol consumption: Excessive

alcohol consumption can have negative effects on both physical and mental health. It can increase the risk of liver disease, cancer, and mental health disorders. Individuals should limit their alcohol consumption to no more than one drink per day for women and two drinks per day for men.

Quit smoking: Smoking is a leading cause of preventable deaths worldwide. It increases the risk of numerous health conditions, including lung cancer, heart disease, and stroke. Quitting smoking is one of the most important things individuals can do to improve their overall health and reduce their risk of chronic diseases.

In conclusion, living a healthy lifestyle is essential for achieving optimal health and well-being. It involves making conscious choices about diet, physical activity, sleep, stress management, social connections, alcohol and tobacco use, and regular medical care. By incorporating healthy habits into daily life, individuals can reduce the risk of chronic diseases and improve their quality of life. It is never too late to start living a healthy lifestyle. Even small changes can make a significant difference in overall health and well-being. It is important to set realistic goals, seek support, and stay committed to making healthy choices every day.

Practice safe sex: Practicing safe sex is essential for protecting against sexually transmitted infections (STIs) and unwanted pregnancies. Individuals should use condoms or other forms of contraception to reduce the risk of STIs and unwanted pregnancies.

Eat a balanced diet: Eating a balanced diet is essential for maintaining good health. It involves consuming a variety of nutrient-dense foods, including fruits, vegetables, whole grains, lean proteins, and healthy fats. Eating a balanced diet can help individuals maintain a healthy weight, reduce the risk of chronic diseases, and improve overall health.

Maintain social connections: Social connections are important for overall health and well-being. They can help individuals reduce stress, improve mood, and provide a sense of purpose and belonging. Individuals should make time for social activities and maintain connections with friends and family members.

Stay up to date with medical check-ups:

Regular medical check-ups can help individuals stay up to date with their health and catch any potential health problems early. It is important to schedule regular check-ups with a healthcare provider and stay up to date with recommended screenings and vaccinations.

Living a healthy lifestyle is not always easy, and it can be challenging to make healthy choices every day. However, by taking small steps and making conscious choices, individuals can improve their overall health and well-being. It is important to stay committed to making healthy choices and seek support when needed. With time and consistency, individuals can live a healthy, happy, and fulfilling life.

Manage chronic conditions: Individuals with chronic conditions, such as diabetes or high blood pressure, should work with their healthcare provider to manage their condition and maintain optimal health. This may involve taking medications as prescribed, monitoring blood sugar or blood pressure levels, and making lifestyle modifications.

Avoid processed and junk food: Processed and junk food are high in calories, unhealthy fats, sugar, and sodium. These foods can contribute to weight gain, inflammation, and chronic diseases. Individuals should limit their consumption of processed and junk food and focus on nutrient-dense whole foods instead.

Find ways to stay active: Physical activity doesn't have to be limited to the gym or structured exercise. Finding ways to incorporate physical activity into daily life, such as taking the stairs instead of the elevator or going for a walk during lunch breaks, can help individuals maintain an active lifestyle and improve overall health.

Practice good hygiene: Good hygiene habits, such as washing hands regularly, brushing and flossing teeth daily, and showering regularly, can help prevent the spread of illness and disease.

Practice safe driving: Safe driving habits, such as wearing a seatbelt, avoiding distracted driving, and obeying traffic laws, can help reduce the risk of car accidents and injuries.

Stay mentally stimulated: Engaging in mentally stimulating activities, such as reading, doing puzzles, or learning a new skill, can help improve cognitive function and reduce the risk of cognitive decline.

Living a healthy lifestyle is a lifelong journey that requires commitment, patience, and consistency. By incorporating healthy habits into daily life, individuals can improve their overall health and reduce the risk of chronic diseases. It is important to set realistic goals, seek support, and stay committed to making healthy choices every day. With time and effort, individuals can achieve optimal health and well-being.